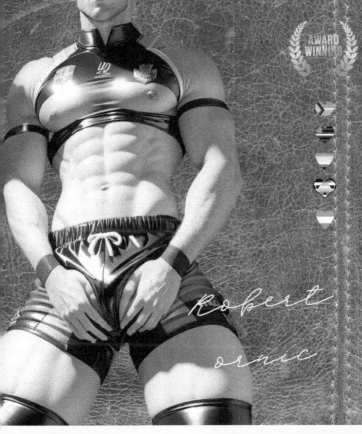

COU

CULTURE

Robert

ornic

Disclaimer:

This book is intended for academic and informational purposes only. It is not meant to stereotype or marginalize any individual or group. The author recognizes and respects the diversity of experiences within the LGBTQ+ community and has made every effort to present these histories with accuracy and sensitivity.

978-1-4467-9782-2

COUNTER CULTURE

For those who have walked before us, showing the way with courage and pride. This book is dedicated to all the brave individuals who fought for acceptance and understanding, enabling the stories shared in these pages to be told.

In the annals of human history, sexuality stands as a pillar of our personal identities and societal norms. The intricate dance of desire and expression, intimacy and display, spans the diverse spectrum of human experience.

We are here to explore a particular facet of this rich tapestry: the history of gay fetish culture, a realm often relegated to the shadows, yet intrinsically tied to the broader narrative of sexuality.

Just as a prism refracts light into a multitude of colours, so too does human sexuality break down into myriad expressions and experiences. Fetish culture, a colorful manifestation of this spectrum, has played an integral role in the formation and evolution of gay identities. Entwined with the tale of gay rights and liberation, fetishism has served as both a covert language of desire and a vehicle of personal liberation.

From ancient times, when same-sex attraction itself was the

transgressive fetish, through the clandestine codes of Victorian gentlemen, to the bold visibility of modern Pride parades, the story of gay fetishism is a fascinating journey. Historically, societies have often sought to regulate the expressions of desire, yet the human spirit continually defies these constraints. In the world of gay fetishism, we find an amplification of this defiance, where normative structures are not just subverted, but fetishized, celebrated, and transformed.

The role of fetish culture in shaping and expressing gay identities extends beyond sexual proclivities. It is a social phenomenon, a communicative language of symbols, and a form of aesthetic and erotic art. The appeal of specific clothing, such as leather jackets, sailor uniforms, or even something as ubiquitous as jeans, goes beyond the object itself, transcending into the realm of symbolic and performative allure.

Consider the foot soldier of the Roman legion, his sturdy calves wrapped in strapping leather sandals, marching with his comrades. Was there desire there, hidden beneath the gaze of Mars and Jupiter? Move forward in time to the Victorian gentleman, his gloved hand brushing another's during an afternoon ride. The touch is casual, yet laden with intent, a fetishized hint towards hidden desires.

Fast-forward to the backrooms of bars in 1970s New York City, where men donned leather jackets and motorcycle caps as statements of a new, defiant masculinity. It was in these clandestine spaces that the undercurrents of gay fetish culture began to rise, swirling together the threads of sexuality, identity, and rebellion. The fetishized attire was not just an assertion of desire but also an act of subversion, of claiming space and challenging norms.

In these narratives, we see the thread of fetishism winding through the centuries, binding together experiences across time and space. We see the impact of societal norms and the powerful draw of the taboo, shaping desires into specific objects or practices. The history of gay fetishes is not a story of outliers or the forbidden. Instead, it is an intimate part of our collective history, a testament to the endless variety of human desire and expression.

Each chapter of this story - from the sands of the Roman Colosseum to the bustling streets of the modern Pride parade - holds its unique allure, its particular blend of desire and defiance. It is an ongoing saga, ever-changing and ever-inspiring, a vibrant testament to the human spirit's unyielding pursuit of expression and connection. As we delve into the chapters of this intriguing chronicle, we journey into the heart of what it means to be human, in all our diverse, beautiful complexity.

As our journey unfolds, we plunge into the shadowy recesses of the past, where desires dared not speak their names, but found their expression in a hidden language of fetishism. Here in the hushed corridors of early homosexual histories, fetishes served as codes, lifelines connecting those who otherwise dared not express their desires.

In the heart of the Renaissance, Italy pulsed with an intense life force that combined art, culture, and illicit desires. A notable figure, Leonardo Da Vinci, was known to sketch beautiful young men, their bodies clothed in flowing robes that seemed to fetishize the unspoken desires of their creator. His work was more than mere artistic expression; it was a veiled exploration of homosexual desires, a collection of fetishized images evoking the beauty of the male form.

Meanwhile, across the English Channel, a secretive society thrived, comprising gentlemen of high standing. This was the Molly

House culture of the 18th century, where men gathered for companionship, intimacy, and an escape from the rigid norms of society. Amid the clandestine gatherings, fetishes became encoded expressions of desire - a silk cravat, a stolen glance, the hint of lace at a man's cuff.

The fetishized objects and behaviors helped these men navigate the dangerous waters of their forbidden desires. While the world outside remained oblivious, within the Molly Houses, they crafted an intricate language of longing. Hidden beneath the surface of everyday objects and gestures, gay fetishism thrived, concealed in plain sight.

Turn now to the Far East, to Edo-era Japan, where an entirely different gay subculture bloomed. The Wakashu, or beautiful youths, were the objects of desire for adult men. Here, the fetishized object was the Kabuki theatre, where these Wakashu performed. The stylized makeup, the striking kimonos, the dramatic poses - all combined to create an atmosphere of intense, fetishized desire.

The enduring Kabuki tradition perpetuated a fetish culture that both concealed and revealed homosexual relationships. This provided an avenue for the expression of gay desires, albeit within the bounds of theatrical performance, serving as a mirror to society, reflecting its fears, hopes, and repressed desires.

Meanwhile, in the Ottoman Empire, the tradition of Turkish

baths offered another locus for closeted desires. Amid the steamy air and echoing tiles, men bathed and relaxed together, a social event overlaid with an undercurrent of eroticism. The bathhouse, with its emphasis on physicality and intimate proximity, became a fetishized space for the exploration of same-sex desire.

From the art-laden halls of the Italian Renaissance, through the secretive Molly Houses of England, to the steam-filled bathhouses of the Ottoman Empire, we find a hidden narrative. Through coded behaviors and fetishized objects, gay men found ways to express their desires, to connect, and to explore their identities within the constraints of their societies.

Fetishism thus played a critical role in early homosexual histories, not merely as an erotic aspect, but as a vital tool for identity formation and community building. While society at large might have misunderstood or condemned these men, within their clandestine gatherings, they found understanding, acceptance, and a shared language of desire. The narrative of gay fetishism is, therefore, not just a story of sexual preferences, but of resilience, creativity, and the human quest for connection.

In the ashes of the Second World War, societies across the globe grappled with transformation and chaos. This tumultuous period, rife with seismic shifts in political, social, and cultural norms, created an atmosphere ripe for the birth of a new counter-culture. Here, in the smoky back-rooms of underground bars and in the hidden corners of rebellious youth culture, gay fetishism found new life and forms.

Consider the leather-clad men of the 1950s, their jackets a blatant challenge to the prescribed norms of the time. In the aftermath of the war, the sight of a man in a leather jacket on a motorcycle came to symbolize rebellion and non-conformity. Within the gay community, this potent symbol was co-opted and fetishized, a tangible emblem of a new, defiant form of masculinity.

In the tender care given to these jackets - the meticulous polishing, the careful stitching of patches - we witness the transformation of a garment into a fetishized object. The leather jacket was not merely a piece of clothing; it was a declaration, a symbol of identity, and a beacon, drawing like-minded individuals together.

In tandem with the rising leather subculture, another fetish was gaining traction - the fascination with uniforms. Soldiers returning from the war often kept their uniforms, wearing them long after their service had ended. Within the gay community, the uniform became a symbol of strength and bravery, echoing undertones of same-sex camaraderie from the battleground.

Across the Atlantic, a similar trend was unfolding. The city of London, still recovering from the ravages of war, was alive with an undercurrent of rebellion. In the dimly lit underground clubs, a unique form of expression began to emerge - the Polari language. A secret code spoken primarily by gay men, Polari allowed them to express their desires openly yet covertly. In this linguistic fetishism, we see another form of rebellion, a repudiation of societal norms enforced by language.

Across the globe, the post-war period was a time of significant social upheaval and change, a potent backdrop for the rise of gay fetish subcultures. As symbols of rebellion were adopted and fetishized, a new language of desire began to form. This language, woven into the fabric of jackets, etched into badges of uniforms, and whispered in secret codes, was the clarion call of a burgeoning counter-culture.

Fueled by the spirit of rebellion and the need for connection, the seeds of a visible, expressive gay culture were sown. Thus, the post-war era marked a crucial turning point in the history of gay fetishism - a period of transformation that would shape the trajectory of gay identities for decades to come.

As the currents of change continued to ripple through the mid-twentieth century, one significant shift took the form of a rather scanty piece of swimwear. This chapter brings us to the bright sunlight and cool waters of the beach and pool culture, where Speedos emerged as a fetishized object in the gay community.

Born in the land Down Under in 1928, the Speedo brand was initially known for its durable and innovative swimwear. However, it was not until the 1950s and '60s that this seemingly mundane piece of swimwear began to take on a deeper significance within the gay community.

In the post-war years, as the tides of social liberation began to rise, the beach became a stage for the display and celebration of the human body. The Speedo, with its revealing cut and form-fitting style, was an ideal player in this new theater of flesh and sun. For the gay men of this era, the allure of the Speedo was manifold. It was not just the physical allure of the male form enhanced by this provocative swimwear, but also the tantalizing prospect of public exhibition and voyeurism that it facilitated.

In the simmering heat of summer, the beach became a vibrant social space where gay men could gather, socialize, and express their desires in a semi-public setting. The simple act of donning a Speedo was at once an embrace of body positivity, a flaunting of societal norms, and a subtle signal to others in the know.

As Speedos gained popularity, they started appearing in the imagery of gay culture. The 1980s saw this swimwear becoming an iconic symbol in media, from the covers of gay pulp fiction to the promotional images of queer dance clubs. In these settings, the Speedo was more than just a garment; it was a fetishized object that symbolized sexual liberation, body confidence, and a sense of playful defiance.

Yet, the story of Speedos is not just a tale of sun and skin. It also tells of the struggle for visibility, acceptance, and equality. At a time when gay men were often stereotyped and stigmatized, the simple act of wearing a Speedo in public was a statement of audacity and pride. It was a way of saying, "I am here, I am queer, and I am not ashamed."

Over the decades, the Speedo has maintained its symbolic potency, evolving and adapting to the changing tides of fashion and culture. From the sparkling beaches of Sydney to the vibrant pool parties of Miami, this humble swimwear has made a significant splash in the history of gay fetish culture. The Speedo, once merely a swimsuit, has become a beacon of boldness, a badge of liberation, and an enduring symbol of gay pride.

From the sun-kissed beaches and sparkling pools, our narrative now turns to the adrenaline-pumped stadiums and grassy fields of sports culture. This chapter explores the allure of National Rugby League (NRL) footy shorts, a seemingly ordinary sports attire that has been fetishized within the gay community.

In the realm of sports, rugby stands as a game emblematic of raw physicality and robust masculinity. The men who play this game, from the professional leagues to the local clubs, are often seen as the epitome of male virility. Amidst the sweat, grit, and adrenaline of the game, the footy shorts worn by these athletes have taken on a life of their own in the realm of gay fetishism.

NRL footy shorts, specifically, are designed for function, allowing players the mobility they need while withstanding the intense physical demands of the game. Yet, it's the tight, revealing nature of these shorts, coupled with the context in which they're worn, that has led to their fetishization within the gay community.

The allure of NRL footy shorts lies in their capacity to accentuate the male physique, drawing attention to muscular thighs and the lower torso. But this appeal extends beyond the physical; it's equally rooted in the symbolism associated with the garment. The footy shorts become a fetishized object that evokes notions of athleticism, masculinity, and a certain rough-and-tumble virility associated with the sport of rugby.

In addition, sports such as rugby often serve as a backdrop for homoerotic undertones - the intimate tackles, the shared camaraderie, the locker room banter. These elements contribute to the fetish appeal of NRL footy shorts, overlaying the physical attraction with a layer of imagined narratives and fantasies.

Over time, the NRL footy shorts found their way from the rugby fields into gay culture at large. They became a common sight at gay clubs and Pride parades, worn as a statement of athletic appeal and a nod to the fetishistic attraction. The sight of footy shorts on the dance floor or parade route became a symbol, a declaration of desire rooted in the unique intersection of sports and sexuality.

In the grand narrative of gay fetishes, NRL footy shorts tell a fascinating story. They show how a piece of sports equipment, rooted in the hyper-masculine world of rugby, can be adopted and fetishized within the gay community. This is a testament to the ever-evolving nature of fetish culture, its ability to imbue the everyday with erotic potential, and the power of symbol and narrative in shaping our desires. From the rugby fields to the dance floors, the journey of NRL footy shorts encapsulates the dynamic, complex, and profoundly human nature of gay fetish history.

The 1960s was a decade of contrasts, of intense upheavals and momentous changes. The eruption of social and political movements during this period made it a hotbed of countercultural ferment. As we explore this era, our attention turns to a unique intersection of fetishism and identity formation: the leather and biker culture within the gay community.

Amid the rebellious spirit of the '60s, a new subculture was taking root, pulling inspiration from the rebellious persona of the archetypal biker. In stark opposition to the clean-cut stereotype of the wholesome American man, bikers represented the rugged, the raw, and the rule-breaking. For gay men, the adoption of biker culture and its fetishization of leather offered a powerful means of subverting traditional expectations of masculinity and sexuality.

Central to this subculture was the leather jacket, a garment steeped in connotations of toughness and rebellion. It was, however, more than just a sartorial choice. The act of donning leather was a transformation, an armor against a society that marginalized and stigmatized them. It symbolized a refusal to conform, a bold declaration of identity, and an assertion of sexual freedom.

Alongside the jacket, a range of other leather garments became fetishized. From trousers and vests to boots and gloves, each item came to carry symbolic weight. Together, they comprised a ritualistic attire, worn as much for its psychological impact as its physical allure.

But this culture extended beyond mere clothing. The fascination with bikers also manifested in the veneration of motorcycles themselves, these mechanical beasts standing as symbols of raw power and unbridled freedom. The motorcycle, much like the leather clothing, was not just a physical object, but a fetishized embodiment of a desired persona.

Leather bars, dedicated spaces for these leather-clad men, began to spring up during this period. These dimly-lit establishments were not just venues for socialization and exploration of their fetishes; they were sanctuaries of acceptance and expression. The establishments became integral to the community, fostering a sense of belonging and providing a space for the leather and biker fetish culture to thrive.

This period also saw the rise of organizations like the Satyrs, the first-known gay motorcycle club, founded in Los Angeles in 1954. Such clubs were instrumental in organizing events like "runs," where members would embark on lengthy motorcycle rides. These events, often culminating in campouts, allowed participants to fully immerse themselves in the biker lifestyle and its associated fetishism.

The leather and biker fetishism of the 1960s was a potent response to the period's social turbulence. It demonstrated the power of fetishes to serve not only as a source of erotic pleasure but also as a form of identity expression and community building. The adoption of leather and biker culture was a defiant statement, a rallying cry, and an affirmation of a collective identity that continues to echo in the annals of gay history.

With the intoxicating scent of leather still hanging in the air, we now delve deeper into the bars and clubs of the era - the clandestine havens where a subculture was born and where the seeds of liberation were sown.

In the mid-20th century, bars and clubs were among the few places where gay men could gather, socialize, and express their identities openly. These spaces, often shrouded in secrecy and coded language, offered a refuge from a society that largely shunned them. Fetish bars, in particular, served as important venues where individuals could explore their desires freely, fostering a sense of camaraderie and collective identity.

The leather bars of the era, for instance, were more than just dimly lit taverns. They were a living, breathing microcosm of the leather and biker subculture. Here, men donned in leather from head to toe engaged in rituals of display and recognition, their outfits serving as badges of identity, their interactions tinged with the erotic undercurrents of their fetish. These bars provided a space for individuals to not just engage with their fetishes, but also to connect with others who shared their desires.

But the importance of these fetish bars extended beyond the personal. They were also instrumental in the broader social and political movement for gay rights. As a gathering spot for the community, these spaces became hotbeds of activism. Here, amidst the clink of glasses and the thrum of conversation, strategies were formed, alliances were built, and movements were mobilized.

Fetish bars played a pivotal role in key historical events like the Stonewall riots in 1969. The

Stonewall Inn, a bar in New York's Greenwich Village, was a haven for the city's gay community, including those with various fetishes. When the police raided this establishment, the community fought back, sparking a series of protests that catalyzed the gay liberation movement.

In the wake of Stonewall, fetish bars continued to serve as sites of resistance and mobilization. These establishments were not just places to escape societal judgment; they were bases from which the fight for acceptance and equality was waged. From organizing demonstrations to providing a platform for activist groups, these bars were at the heart of the community's struggle for rights and recognition.

In the narrative of gay history, fetish bars stand as emblematic landmarks. They reflect the intertwined personal and political journeys of a community navigating a hostile social landscape. As sites of desire, identity, and resistance, these establishments highlight the potent role of fetishism in shaping the path towards gay liberation.

Moving from the electric energy of fetish bars, we step into the realm of personal expression and the redefinition of masculinity. Chapter 8 uncovers the emergence of the 'bear' culture and the symbolism of moustaches within the gay community, both powerful elements in challenging traditional notions of masculinity.

In mainstream culture, the 'ideal' man was often depicted as lean and athletic, clean-shaven with a neatly groomed appearance. However, as the gay community explored its identity in the latter half of the 20th century, a counter-narrative emerged. A new archetype, the 'bear', started to gain popularity, representing a subculture that celebrated the natural, rugged man. These men, often larger and hairier with a strikingly visible feature - the moustache, challenged the standard image of male beauty.

'Bears' were unapologetically themselves. They reveled in their burly bodies, their chest and facial hair, and their typically rugged demeanor, a stark contrast to societal expectations. The culture was a celebration of diversity within the gay community, a pushback against both heteronormative standards and the prescriptive masculinity within gay culture itself.

Integral to this new image was the moustache, a potent symbol of masculinity and a defining characteristic of the 'bear'. Across cultures, a moustache has often been associated with virility and manhood. In the context of 'bear' culture, it served as a badge of a specific masculine identity, a visual shorthand for a subculture that prized authenticity and body positivity over conventional attractiveness.

The 'bear' culture was not just a subculture in the shadows; it was a public, vibrant, and influential part of the gay community. 'Bear' events, like the International Mr. Bear Competition, drew participants from around the globe. Similarly, 'bear' bars began to appear, serving as communal spaces for 'bears' and their admirers. 'Bear' magazines, films, and artwork also started to gain prominence, illustrating the extent to which this counter-narrative had permeated the gay cultural landscape.

The emergence of the 'bear' culture and the fetishization of moustaches represent a pivotal moment in gay history. They illustrate how the community began to question, resist, and redefine notions of masculinity.

Through these expressions, gay men created a more inclusive understanding of male beauty and desirability, one that recognized and celebrated a wide range of body types, appearances, and expressions of masculinity. This redefinition of masculinity served not just as a personal affirmation, but as a broader statement about diversity and acceptance within the gay community.

Let us whisk away to the realm of athletic masculinity and the fetishization of a piece of sporting equipment: the jockstrap. This protective garment, initially designed to safeguard male athletes during strenuous physical activity, would come to play an intriguing role in gay fetish culture.

Jockstraps first originated in the late 19th century as a practical response to the growing enthusiasm for cycling in Boston. These devices, originally named "Bike Jockey Straps," were designed to provide support and protection to male cyclists navigating the city's cobblestone streets. Over time, the utility of the jockstrap extended to other sports, becoming a staple in the wardrobe of athletes across a variety of disciplines.

The jockstrap's transition from functional sports gear to a fetishized item within the gay community was a complex process, rooted in the garment's associations with athleticism, masculinity, and the tantalizing promise of what it concealed. The jockstrap's minimalistic design, exposing the wearer's buttocks while cradling their genitals, made it ripe for eroticization. It was this blend of utilitarian purpose and erotic potential that lent the jockstrap its unique allure.

In the realm of gay fetish culture, the jockstrap came to symbolize a potent form of masculine sexuality. The garment was linked to the world of sports, an arena traditionally associated with virility, strength, and masculine camaraderie. Moreover, the jockstrap's design inherently drew attention to the male physique in a manner that was both provocative and tantalizing. It was, in essence, a celebration of male sexuality

Uniforms, tailored with precision, exude an aura of authority and control. Military uniforms, in particular, command respect and admiration due to the values of honor, courage, and strength they symbolize. Throughout history, military uniforms have also woven themselves into the rich tapestry of gay fetish culture, shaping fantasies and fueling desires.

As early as World War II, men in uniform started to become a recurring motif in the collective gay psyche. Thousands of men serving in the military, their youth and vitality framed by their crisp attire, presented an image of masculinity that was both captivating and tantalizing. The close quarters in which these servicemen lived and the camaraderie fostered by the intense conditions of war created a milieu where explorations of sexuality could flourish.

In the 1950s and 1960s, the fetishization of military uniforms became even more pronounced as physique magazines started to feature servicemen on their covers. These publications, operating under the guise of promoting fitness and athleticism, were, in fact, catering to the gay market. Images of chiseled soldiers, sailors, and airmen became staples of these magazines, fueling fantasies and shaping desires within the gay community.

Yet, the allure of military uniforms extended beyond mere aesthetics. The power dynamics inherent in the military hierarchy played a crucial role in their fetishization. The uniforms served as potent symbols of authority and dominance, invoking fantasies of discipline and submission. On the other hand, they also prompted narratives of resistance and rebellion against the structures of power they represented.

This dynamic was further complicated by the military's historical hostility towards homosexuality. The uniforms, thus, became emblematic of a forbidden desire, amplifying their erotic appeal. Wearing a military uniform or engaging in role-play allowed gay men to not only explore these dynamics of power and desire but also to subvert an institution that had often marginalized them.

With the advent of the internet and the digital age, military fetishism found new avenues for expression and exploration. Online platforms and communities dedicated to the fetish emerged, allowing individuals across the globe to share their fantasies and experiences.

Today, the military uniform continues to hold sway in the realm of gay fetish culture. It represents a complex interplay of power, authority, resistance, and desire. It remains a potent symbol, a fabric woven with threads of history and desire, stitched into the rich, diverse quilt of gay fetish culture.

As we shift our gaze back to the sporting realm, we find ourselves entranced by a singular piece of attire: the jockstrap. Unlike the broad swath of fabric that forms a military uniform, a jockstrap is a study in minimalism. Designed originally for utility on the sports field, it became an object of erotic fascination within the gay community, its allure woven into the fabric of gay fetish culture.

The jockstrap first stepped onto the scene in the late 19th century, designed as a practical solution for bicycle jockeys navigating the uneven cobblestones of Boston. Yet, as the garment found its place in various sports, it began to transcend its utilitarian purpose. Its scant design, offering support to the genitals while leaving the buttocks exposed, added an erotic edge to its functionality.

Within the gay community, the jockstrap became a tantalizing spectacle. Here was a garment that veered towards the audacious, highlighting and accentuating male sexuality. The jockstrap's direct association with sports—an arena often characterized by raw energy, physical prowess, and male camaraderie—bolstered its erotic appeal.

In the confines of gay bars, clubs, and private parties, men adorned in jockstraps became a common sight. The garment offered a way to flirt with exposure, to provoke and titillate, while hinting at the athletic and masculine. It was a bold statement of sexual confidence, a nod to the sporting world, and a symbol of erotic freedom all at once.

Over the years, the jockstrap has retained its popularity within the gay fetish culture. From its inception as a protective gear for cyclists to its present-day status as an erotic symbol, the jockstrap has journeyed through history, earning its place in the annals of gay fetishism. Even today, whether on the pages of a gay erotica novel or in the dim light of a gay club, the jockstrap continues to command attention, its minimalistic design and sporting heritage fueling fantasies and shaping desires.

The veil lifts from the world of BDSM - bondage, discipline, dominance, submission, sadism, and masochism - as we delve into Chapter 11. The world of BDSM isn't just an obscure corner of sexual exploration; it's an arena where power dynamics are played out and consent is held supreme. Within the spectrum of gay fetishism, BDSM practices have found a prominent place, creating spaces where individuals could push boundaries and explore aspects of their sexuality in a controlled, consensual environment.

As early as the 1950s, hints of BDSM practices started to appear in the burgeoning gay fetish culture. Gay men began exploring power dynamics through their sexual encounters, with some taking on dominant roles and others reveling in submission. Leather culture, in particular, began to incorporate elements of BDSM, with leather bars serving as spaces where these practices could be explored safely and consensually.

As the years rolled on, the BDSM culture within the gay community began to evolve. BDSM wasn't just about the exchange of power; it was also about trust, communication, and mutual respect. The dominant partner, often called the 'Top' or 'Dom', held the power to control the scene, but this power was given willingly by the submissive partner, the 'Bottom' or 'Sub'. The practice of 'safe words' was introduced to ensure that the scene could be stopped at any point should the Sub feel uncomfortable.

BDSM practices started to spill over into the broader culture of gay fetishes. The image of a man in a leather harness, for instance, was as much a BDSM symbol as it was a symbol of gay fetishism. Role-play scenarios involving elements of BDSM also began to gain popularity, adding another layer of depth to the world of gay fetishes.

BDSM events, like Folsom Street Fair in San Francisco or MAL (Mid-Atlantic Leather) in Washington, D.C., began to emerge, attracting thousands of participants from the gay community and beyond. These events served as a celebration of kink culture, providing safe spaces where individuals could express their fetishes openly and proudly.

From its early days to the present, the intersection of BDSM and gay fetishism has offered a space for exploration, discovery, and self-expression. The world of BDSM is more than whips and chains; it's a realm where individuals can explore power, control, and submission in a consensual and safe manner. It's a testament to the diversity of human sexuality and the myriad ways it can be expressed and experienced.

In the annals of the human experience, the invention of the internet will forever be etched as a pivotal turning point, a revolution that touched all aspects of life, including the exploration and expression of sexuality. In the realm of gay fetishism, the internet emerged not only as a tool for connection and communication but also as a vast, virtual landscape ripe for exploration and discovery.

During the internet's early years, online forums and chat rooms became havens for the LGBTQ+ community, offering safe spaces for individuals to communicate, share experiences, and build a sense of community. Fetish-specific sites began to appear, providing platforms for individuals with specific kinks to connect with like-minded others. This virtual landscape offered an anonymity that allowed many to explore their fetishes without fear of judgment or stigma.

As technology evolved, so did these online spaces. Interactive websites, online video platforms, and eventually social media gave individuals new ways to explore and express their fetishes. Photos, videos, and live streams brought fetish culture to life in the virtual realm, enabling individuals to visually share their experiences and engage in online role-play.

Digital platforms also proved instrumental in the proliferation of fetish-related information. From educational websites dedicated to safe BDSM practices to blogs exploring the history and evolution of various fetishes, the internet became a treasure trove of information for both the curious and the experienced.

Online communities began to emerge around specific fetishes, providing support, guidance, and a sense of belonging to their members. These communities were not just confined to local or regional areas; they spanned across borders, connecting individuals globally.

The rise of the internet also impacted the commercial aspect of gay fetishism. Online stores selling fetish gear sprang up, offering a wide range of products from leather harnesses to jockstraps. The internet also made fetish events more accessible, with details of local and international events easily available at one's fingertips.

With the rise of the internet, the world of gay fetishism expanded exponentially, creating a digital landscape as diverse and complex as the one in the physical world. It is a testament to the profound impact of technology on human sexuality, reflecting our innate desire to connect, explore, and express our most intimate selves.

Now we will immerses ourselves in the visually captivating world of fetish photography and art within the gay culture. This art form, vibrant and bold, has not only served as a vehicle for expression but also has been instrumental in documenting the evolution of gay fetishism over the years.

Our journey begins in the mid-20th century with the emergence of physique photography. Riding the wave of post-war liberation, magazines like Physique Pictorial began featuring athletic men in various states of undress, often posing with props suggestive of different fetishes. Though operating under the guise of promoting fitness, these magazines catered to a predominantly gay audience, serving up tantalizing images of male beauty and masculinity.

Among the most influential figures in this era was Touko Laaksonen, better known by his pseudonym Tom of Finland. His hyper-masculine drawings, brimming with leather-clad, muscle-bound men, presented a bold, unapologetic depiction of gay fetishism. His work challenged the contemporary, often negative, stereotypes of gay men, instead showcasing them as confident, strong, and sexually empowered.

As we advance into the 1970s and 80s, fetish photography and art took a turn towards the explicit. Artists like Robert Mapplethorpe pushed the boundaries with their provocative imagery, often featuring leather, BDSM, and other fetish elements. Despite facing controversy and criticism, these artists played a crucial role in bringing fetish art into the mainstream discourse, prompting conversations around sexual freedom, consent, and artistic expression.

With the dawn of the digital age, the landscape of fetish photography and art underwent a significant transformation. Artists and photographers found new platforms to showcase their work, reaching a global audience with the click of a button. Social media platforms, online galleries, and digital magazines now host a multitude of fetish-inspired artworks, reflecting the diversity of gay fetish culture.

Through the lens of fetish photography and art, we witness the evolution of gay fetish culture, from the coy physique magazines of the 50s to the bold, unapologetic imagery of the digital age. This art form has not only documented the changing face of fetishism but has also played a critical role in challenging societal norms, breaking taboos, and advocating for sexual freedom and expression. In a world often too eager to judge, fetish photography and art offer a defiant celebration of desire, diversity, and the human body.

T hroughout the years, the
media, in its various forms,
has shaped and reflected
societal attitudes towards
sexuality. Gay fetishism, long
relegated to the shadows,
gradually found its way onto
screens large and small, fostering

visibility, understanding, and sometimes controversy.

The first glimmers of gay fetish representation can be traced back to the mid-20th century, a time when the constraints of censorship and societal attitudes kept depictions of homosexuality, let alone fetishism, mostly hidden. However, subtly coded characters and narratives started to emerge, hinting at a broader spectrum of sexuality.

By the 1970s and 80s, film and television began to push boundaries. Directors such as Rainer Werner Fassbinder and Pedro Almodóvar presented films that not only openly depicted homosexuality but also delved into various facets of gay fetish culture. These films, often provocative and controversial, brought to light a subculture that had been largely kept hidden, presenting complex narratives of desire, identity, and sexuality.

Television, initially slower in its approach, gradually followed suit. Shows like "Queer as Folk" and "The L Word" included characters and narratives that explored different fetishes. These shows not only entertained audiences but also opened a dialogue about sexuality, diversity, and acceptance.

Into the 21st century, the growth of streaming platforms led to a proliferation of LGBTQ+ content, including narratives that delved into fetish culture. Series like "Bonding" explored the world of BDSM through a comedic lens, while others took a more dramatic approach. The medium's ability to depict multifaceted characters and intricate story arcs allowed for a deeper exploration of gay fetish culture.

Media's influence on the visibility and understanding of gay fetishism cannot be underestimated. As films and TV shows started depicting fetishes more openly, they reflected and contributed to a cultural shift towards acceptance. Yet, representation remains a double-edged sword, with media also criticized for perpetuating stereotypes and sensationalizing fetishism.

As the line between the mainstream and the marginal continues to blur, media's role in shaping our understanding of gay fetishism becomes increasingly vital. As the lens focuses and refocuses, the portrayal of gay fetishism on screen continues to evolve, contributing to a broader, more nuanced dialogue about sexuality, desire, and identity.

W e will now look through the chic lanes of queer fashion, where tight jeans, crop tops, and an array of other trends serve as both personal expressions of style and significant signifiers within the history of gay fetishism.

Tight jeans, for instance, aren't merely a fashion statement. Their rise in popularity among gay men in the 70s and 80s mirrored the growing sexual liberation within the community. Tight jeans showcased the male form in a way that was both casual and provocative, a symbol of rebellion against the constraints of traditional masculinity.

Crop tops, too, occupy an essential place in queer fashion history. In the 1980s, men sporting crop tops became a common sight within the gay community, with this trend reaching its zenith in the mid-80s when stars like Prince and Freddie Mercury donned them on stage. These garments defied gender norms, allowing men to embrace a traditionally feminine article of clothing while simultaneously accentuating their physique.

Leather, as discussed in previous chapters, has been a potent symbol within the gay fetish scene. The evolution of leather fashion - from biker jackets and vests to harnesses and chaps - underscores the growing visibility and acceptance of gay fetishism. What began as a niche interest within the gay biker culture transformed into a global phenomenon, transcending its subcultural origins to influence mainstream fashion.

As we venture into the 21st century, queer fashion continues to evolve and intersect with gay fetishism. Brands and designers, from high-end fashion houses to independent queer labels, have embraced and incorporated fetish-inspired elements into their collections. Materials such as latex, PVC, and mesh, along with styles reminiscent of BDSM wear, have found their way onto fashion runways and city streets.

Moreover, the advent of the internet and social media has democratized fashion, making queer and fetish-inspired trends more accessible. Platforms like Instagram have become virtual runways, showcasing a diverse range of queer fashion and promoting body positivity and self-expression.

The exploration of queer fashion reveals it to be much more than an array of trends; it's a narrative of the gay community's history, a reflection of shifting societal attitudes, and a bold expression of identity and desire. As we continue to trace the contours of this ever-evolving landscape, it becomes clear that the interplay between fashion and gay fetishism is not just about aesthetics; it's an integral part of the cultural fabric of the queer community.

n the stimulating realm of gay fetishism, we will dive into the intriguing world of rubber and latex subcultures. These glossy, skin-tight materials have, over the decades, formed a distinct niche within the LGBTQ+ community, their allure rooted in a blend of aesthetics, sensory experience, and symbolism.

The fascination with rubber and latex has its origins in the mid-20th century. The post-war boom saw these materials gain popularity due to their widespread use in industry and consumer goods. Within the gay community, they started to gain a following among individuals who found the tactile sensation of wearing rubber or latex arousively unique and visually striking.

By the 1980s and 90s, with the increasing visibility of the BDSM community, the rubber and latex fetishes had solidified their presence in gay culture. These materials became synonymous with BDSM practices, with their shiny, body-conforming attributes accentuating the wearer's physique, while also reflecting themes of control and submission often associated with BDSM.

The appeal of rubber and latex extends beyond their visual and tactile aspects. For many enthusiasts, the act of wearing these materials transforms into an immersive experience. The tight fit of latex and rubber clothing creates a sensation of a second skin, an intimate, enclosing embrace that many describe as uniquely comforting or exciting.

Rubber and latex subcultures have their rituals, norms, and events. 'Rubbermen' and 'latex lovers' gather at dedicated club nights and events, such as Mister

International Rubber in Chicago or Folsom Street Fair in San Francisco, where the community's camaraderie comes alive amidst a sea of gleaming bodies. These events provide a safe and accepting environment for individuals to explore their fetish, make connections, and celebrate their shared interests.

As we journey through the 21st century, the rubber and latex subcultures continue to evolve, propelled by advancements in materials, design, and the growing mainstream acceptance of fetish culture. These developments have seen a rise in the diversity of latex and rubber clothing available, from the traditional catsuits and masks to more everyday wearable pieces.

The exploration of rubber and latex subcultures in this chapter offers a unique glimpse into the diverse spectrum of gay fetishism. It underlines the importance of community, acceptance, and the freedom to explore one's desires in an environment of respect and consent. The story of rubber and latex fetishism is not just about a specific material preference, but a testament to the human capacity for sexual diversity and expression.

We now embark on an exploration of an especially distinctive realm within the spectrum of gay fetishism: puppy play. This form of role-play, in which participants adopt the characteristics of a canine and its handler, embodies a fascinating mix of comfort, freedom, and power dynamics.

Puppy play, though seemingly a contemporary phenomenon, can trace its roots to the earlier manifestations of animal role-play in the BDSM community. However, it has carved out its own unique space, differentiating itself through a focus on the playful, affectionate, and non-aggressive attributes of canine behavior.

Participants in puppy play, often referred to as 'pups' or 'dogs', adopt the persona of their chosen role, donning accessories such as pup hoods, collars, and even mitts designed to mimic paws. Handlers, on the other hand, guide their pups, providing structure, rewards, and sometimes discipline. The dynamic is often one of care and guidance rather than domination and submission, differing significantly from conventional perceptions of BDSM.

This form of role-play offers individuals a chance to shed their human concerns and inhibitions. For pups, it can provide a sense of freedom, allowing them to tap into a simpler, more instinctual state of mind. For handlers, it often fulfills a nurturing instinct, giving them a role of responsibility and control.

Within the gay community, puppy play has flourished into a subculture with its own codes of behavior, communities, and events. 'Pup packs', or groups of like-minded enthusiasts, have formed both online and offline, providing supportive spaces for individuals to learn, share experiences, and make connections. Major cities around the world host 'Pup Mosh' events, where pups and handlers can meet, play, and compete in a safe and welcoming environment.

Despite its unconventional nature, puppy play has gained more visibility and acceptance in recent years, breaking into mainstream consciousness through popular media and discussions around sexual diversity. This subculture underscores the broad and intricate variety within gay fetishism, emphasizing that, beyond mere sexual gratification, these practices often fulfill deeper emotional and psychological needs. The exploration of puppy play reaffirms that human sexuality is complex, diverse, and resoundingly unique.

Our focus now shifts towards the vibrant, colourful world of Pride parades, a global phenomenon that encapsulates the LGBTQ+ community's spirit, diversity, and defiance. These public celebrations provide a platform for individuals to openly express their sexual identities, including the display of fetishes and kinks, leading to a visible and significant representation of gay fetishism.

Originating in the wake of the Stonewall Riots of 1969 as a potent symbol of resistance and visibility, Pride parades have evolved to become inclusive celebrations of LGBTQ+ identities. As they've grown more widespread and mainstream, these parades have offered the opportunity for various subgroups within the queer community, including those involved in fetish and kink, to gain visibility and acceptance.

Pride parades have become a canvas for the flamboyant display of fetishes. Participants don leather, latex, harnesses, pup hoods, military uniforms, and other fetish-inspired outfits, transforming the streets into a vibrant tableau of sexual diversity. These displays serve as an assertion of the community's presence and a celebration of sexual freedom and expression.

However, the public display of fetishes at Pride parades is not without controversy. Critics argue that such explicit displays could reinforce negative stereotypes about the LGBTQ+ community, or that they may not be appropriate for all attendees, including families and children. Advocates counter that these displays are crucial for promoting visibility and acceptance of the full range of queer identities and experiences.

The presence of fetishes at Pride parades also highlights the intersections between sexuality, politics, and public space. By openly expressing their kinks and fetishes, participants challenge societal norms and expectations about what is considered 'acceptable' or 'appropriate'. These displays, often provocative and rebellious, contribute to a broader dialogue about sexual freedom, consent, and diversity.

As we navigate the 21st century, Pride parades continue to evolve, reflecting the changing landscape of queer identities and experiences. The visible presence of fetishes and kinks at these events underscores their role as platforms for liberation and acceptance, venues where the full spectrum of queer life can be openly and proudly displayed. By challenging norms and pushing boundaries, Pride parades serve as a vibrant, vital testament to the diversity and resilience of the LGBTQ+ community.

Time for a closer look at the journey of one particularly emblematic piece of attire from the fetish scene to the mainstream fashion world: the harness. This item, once exclusively associated with BDSM and leather subcultures, has undergone a fascinating transformation, its history reflecting broader changes within gay culture and society as a whole.

The origins of the harness within gay fetishism are linked to the post-World War II period, particularly within the leather and biker subcultures. These groups appropriated the harness, initially used for practical purposes in fields like construction and climbing, and integrated it into their aesthetic. The harness was embraced for its ability to accentuate the male form, imbuing the wearer with a sense of power and virility. Moreover, it was laden with symbolism, its associations with control and bondage resonating within BDSM practices.

Over the decades, the harness remained a powerful symbol within the gay fetish scene. Its presence at events like Pride parades and fetish parties, as well as its depiction in queer art and media, reinforced its status as a signifier of rebellion, non-conformity, and sexual liberation.

However, the turn of the 21st century marked the beginning of a surprising evolution for the harness. As societal attitudes towards homosexuality and fetishism began to shift, elements of these subcultures began to infiltrate the mainstream, the harness among them.

Fashion designers began incorporating harnesses into their collections, interpreting this fetish item in new and innovative ways.

What began as an underground symbol of kink started appearing on high-fashion runways, worn by models and celebrities, and featured in popular fashion magazines.

The harness's journey from fetish to mainstream underscores the reciprocal influence between subcultures and popular culture. It showcases how symbols of sexual subversion can be reinterpreted and repurposed, contributing to a broader societal conversation about sexuality, expression, and norms.

Nevertheless, as the harness gains mainstream acceptance, questions of appropriation and sanitization arise. Some argue that its incorporation into mainstream fashion dilutes its original meaning and symbolism, while others view it as a positive step towards greater visibility and acceptance of queer culture.

The story of the harness serves as a microcosm of the evolving relationship between gay fetishism and society, illustrating how these interactions are never static, always reflecting the fluidity and complexity of human sexuality.

The AIDS crisis of the 1980s, and its profound impact on the gay community, including those engaged in fetish and kink practices. This period marked a significant shift in attitudes and behaviors, as fear, stigma, and grief swept across the community.

The emergence of AIDS introduced a chilling new reality for gay men. A sense of fear and uncertainty permeated the community, impacting not just physical health but mental and emotional well-being. Within the context of fetish and kink, practices that once provided a source of freedom, joy, and connection were now tinged with anxiety.

Amidst the height of the crisis, the gay fetish community faced additional layers of stigma. Fetish and kink practices were often misrepresented in mainstream media, further perpetuating harmful stereotypes about promiscuity and risk. This added to the already prevalent homophobia, complicating the community's response to the crisis.

However, in the face of adversity, the fetish and kink community demonstrated resilience and adaptability. A profound sense of camaraderie and collective responsibility emerged. Community-led initiatives focused on education and safer-sex practices sprang up, aiming to protect members while maintaining the essence of their sexual expression. New codes of behavior were established, prioritizing consent, communication, and safety.

The leather community, for instance, played a crucial role in AIDS activism and relief efforts.

Leather clubs and bars became hubs for fundraising and awareness campaigns, contributing significantly to organizations like the AIDS Memorial Quilt project. Leaders within the leather community used their influence to educate about safe sex practices, effectively slowing the rate of infection within their circles.

The impact of the AIDS crisis on the fetish and kink community is a testament to the capacity of human beings to adapt and persevere in the face of overwhelming adversity. It highlights the role of community in navigating crises, providing support, and effecting change.

The AIDS crisis inevitably left an indelible mark on the history of gay fetishism. It forced a reevaluation of practices, fueled a shift towards safer sex practices, and engendered a generation of activists. Despite the heartrending losses, the crisis ultimately forged a stronger, more health-conscious community, resilient in the face of adversity and committed to the well-being of its members.

As we enter the penultimate chapter, we consider the future trajectory of gay fetishes. The social landscape has witnessed remarkable transformations over the past decades, changing perceptions around homosexuality and fetishism. But what lies ahead? In Chapter 21, we speculate on the shifting boundaries, evolving perceptions, and potential trajectories of gay fetish culture.

A more accepting social environment, coupled with greater visibility of queer identities, has led to an increased normalization of gay fetishes. The advent of the internet has played a crucial role in this shift. Online platforms provide safe spaces for individuals to explore their desires, learn, and connect with like-minded people, pushing the boundaries of acceptance and understanding.

As society becomes more sex-positive, there is likely to be an increased recognition of the diversity of human sexuality, including fetishes. The once clear lines that separated the 'normal' from the 'deviant' are blurring. However, this openness to diversity raises questions about the future identity of gay fetishism. As these practices gain mainstream acceptance, will they retain their status as fetishes, or will they evolve into merely another facet of human sexual expression?

Despite increased acceptance, it is also important to consider the potential for backlash. Societal attitudes can shift in both directions, and progress is rarely linear. Increased visibility may also lead to greater scrutiny, misrepresentation, and commodification, challenging the community's autonomy and authentic self-expression.

On a more optimistic note, the future could see an increased emphasis on education around fetishes and kink. Already, we see initiatives within the fetish community focused on promoting informed consent, safety, and communication. As society becomes more open to these practices, there may be a shift towards more comprehensive sex education, encompassing the wide spectrum of human desire.

Looking ahead, it is clear that the future of gay fetishes is not set in stone. It will continue to evolve and adapt, shaped by societal attitudes, technological advancements, and the ever-changing landscape of the gay community itself. Whatever the future holds, the history of gay fetishism serves as a testament to the diversity and resilience of human sexuality, reminding us of the extraordinary capacity for change and adaptation.

Throughout this journey, we've traced the trajectory of gay fetishism from the clandestine shadows of societal disapproval to the vibrant, increasingly accepted facet of human sexuality it is today. This path has not been a smooth or linear one, but rather a multifaceted and complex evolution, shaped by historical events, social progress, and internal community dynamics.

In the face of adversity, including criminalization, social stigma, and the devastating impact of the AIDS crisis, the gay fetish community has demonstrated an inspiring resilience. Its members have consistently pushed the boundaries of societal norms, fought for their rights to pleasure and self-expression, and forged spaces, both physical and virtual, where they can celebrate their desires.

We've also observed the fascinating interplay between the gay fetish community and mainstream culture. Elements of fetish culture have permeated the broader social consciousness, influencing fashion, art, and popular perceptions of sexuality. Yet, even as some elements of gay fetish culture gain mainstream acceptance, the community continues to evolve and diversify, reflecting the inherently fluid nature of human desire.

Moving forward, the path is not fully charted. The internet and evolving social attitudes offer both opportunities and challenges for the gay fetish community. As this culture becomes more visible and accepted, it is crucial to ensure that this does not lead to commodification or erasure of its rich history and significance.

This book is not an endpoint but an invitation for further

exploration, understanding, and discussion. The history of gay fetish culture is a living, evolving narrative, one that is being continuously written by its community members. As we look to the future, the continuing evolution of gay fetish culture reminds us of the boundless diversity of human sexuality and the enduring power of desire.

Milton Keynes UK
Ingram Content Group UK Ltd.
UKHW040628280723
425958UK00001B/8